OXR

GW00372451

Transport Statistics Report

Car and Driver Injury Accident and Casualty Rates
Great Britain: 1990

April 1992

London: HMSO

Prepared for publication by STD5 branch
Directorate of Statistics
Department of Transport

Derek Jones
Alfred Munster

GOVERNMENT STATISTICAL SERVICE

A service of statistical information and advice is provided to the government by specialist staff employed in the statistics divisions of individual Departments. Statistics are made generally available through their publications and further information and advice on them can be obtained from the Departments concerned.

Enquiries about the contents of this publication should be made to:

Directorate of Statistics
Department of Transport
Room B6.49
Romney House
43 Marsham Street
London
SW1P 3PY

Telephone 071-276 8780

Produced from Camera Ready Copy supplied by the department.

The price of this publication has been set to make some contribution to the preparation cost incurred at the Department of Transport.

Printed in the United Kingdom for HMSO
Dd294973 3/92 C8 G3390 10170

CONTENTS	Page

Commentary

1. Introduction   1

2. Coverage   1

3. Use and interpretation of results   2

4. Results   4

Definitions   7

Section 1: Injury accident involvement and casualty rates

Table 1: Rates of involvement in injury accidents:
by size of car and ownership: 1990   9

Table 2: Car user casualty rates:
by size of car and ownership: 1990   10

Table 3: Rates of involvement in injury accidents:
by make/model and ownership: 1990   11

Table 4: Car user casualty rates:
by make/model and ownership: 1990   14

Section 2: Risk of injury to drivers involved in injury accidents

Table 5: Risk of injury to drivers involved in injury accidents:
by various factors: 1989-90   17

Table 6: Risk of injury to drivers involved in injury accidents:
by make/model: 1989-90   18

**Appendix 1: Information on car mileage drawn from the
National Travel Survey 1985/6**   20

Appendix 2: Explanatory notes to statistical analyses   21

COMMENTARY

1. Introduction

By agreement between the Department of Transport and police forces throughout Great Britain, details of all road accidents reported to the police in which a person is injured are transmitted to the Department of Transport in the form of a standard report (STATS19), usually through the appropriate local authority. These accident reports provide the basis for the Department's work on monitoring and analysis of road accident statistics.

From January 1989 the standard report prepared by the police was modified to include the registration marks of all motor vehicles involved. By linking the registration marks with the vehicle data held by the Driver and Vehicle Licensing Agency (DVLA) at Swansea, a range of extra information about the vehicles involved in injury accidents can now be obtained. No personal details, such as names or addresses, are collected in this process.

This is the second report of results based on these additional vehicle data. It compares the injury accident records of different types and models of car and the types and numbers of casualties resulting. The first report of this type, covering accidents in 1989, was published by HMSO in May 1991.

This report is similar in scope to the 1989 edition but is presented in a different format. Tables are presented in two sections. The tables in Section 1 deal with rates of involvement in injury accidents and casualty rates per 10,000 licensed vehicles during the year 1990. Those in Section 2 deal with the risks of injury to drivers involved in injury accidents during 1989 and 1990, and benefit from a more detailed statistical analysis of the influences on driver injury risk than the corresponding tables in the 1989 report.

2. Coverage

It is not possible to link all vehicles involved in road injury accidents with data at DVLA. Details of foreign, diplomatic and military vehicles and those with trade plates are not held at DVLA. In addition, registration marks are generally unavailable for vehicles which leave the scene of an accident and some registration marks which appear to have a valid format prove untraceable. Remaining technical problems resulted in a few police forces and local authorities not submitting registration marks.

In 1990 these factors collectively resulted in roughly 20 percent of vehicles having no additional vehicle details. However, any bias due to the missing data is unlikely to significantly influence the results tabulated. The 80 percent of available data are sufficient to allow estimates of accident rate to be made by size, age and type of ownership of car. Where the number of licensed cars is sufficiently large, rates have also been calculated for individual models of car.

The rates in Section 1 are per 10,000 licensed vehicles as recorded by the Annual Vehicle Census carried out in December 1990. However, it has been estimated that about $3\frac{1}{2}$ percent of cars in use are unlicensed. Some of these cars will have been involved in accidents, although they tend to be older and have lower annual mileages. They are unlikely to distort comparisons between different groups of cars significantly.

The tables in Section 2, which present the percentage of drivers that are injured once involved in an injury accident, make use of all data collected during 1989 as well as 1990. This has allowed larger sample sizes and a consequent increase in the reliability of the results.

3. Use and interpretation of results

3.1. Exposure

Road accidents and the casualties that result from them depend on many factors, of which driver behaviour is the most important. Other principal factors include the road environment and condition, and the vehicle type and condition.

In addition to these factors, the number of road injury accidents involving a particular type of vehicle will depend on the number of such vehicles on the road and the average mileage driven. These influences are known collectively as measures of exposure.

The Department obtains information on vehicle populations through analysis of DVLA registrations data. The accident involvement and car user casualty rates in Section 1 are given per 10,000 licensed vehicles in each group. General information on the drivers and average mileage covered by different types, but not models, of car is available from the National Travel Survey, and is summarised in Appendix 1.

3.2. Primary and secondary safety

The role of the vehicle and its driver can be considered in two parts; the degree to which the driver and vehicle influence the risk of accidents, and the degree to which, once involved in an accident, the vehicle prevents injury to its occupants and other persons involved.

The risk of being involved in accidents is influenced mainly by driver behaviour, because the vast majority of accidents are initiated by driver error. However, vehicle characteristics such as braking, handling, lighting and drivers' fields of vision, known as primary safety factors, can influence the effects of driver error on accident risk, as can the road and traffic management infrastructure.

Once involved in accidents, the number of injuries and their severity also depend on several factors. However in this case, the inherent protection offered by the vehicle to its occupants, especially the driver, is probably the most important influence on the safety record of the car. Factors that influence this are known as secondary safety factors. The design of the car body is crucial to determining how crash energy is absorbed and the degree of intrusion into the passenger compartment. Also very important are the design of the seat-belts, steering wheel and column and other interior fittings such as energy absorbing material in the dash-board, doors and other areas which occupants might contact in a crash. Other safety features such as air bags and pre-tensioned seat-belts further reduce injury risk. Important non-vehicle factors include impact speed and direction and type of object struck, which are influenced by driver behaviour and usage patterns, for example the proportion of urban driving.

3.3. Description of tables

Section 1: Injury accident involvement and casualty rates

Tables 1 and 3 show the extent to which drivers and their cars become involved in injury accidents. This is influenced mainly by driver behaviour, average mileage and pattern of use. The safety characteristics of the car will also have some influence but this is difficult to assess. Tables 2 and 4 show car user casualty rates, which are influenced by the combined effects of accident involvement, accident type, the number of passengers and secondary safety features.

Table 1 shows rates of involvement in injury accidents per 10,000 licensed vehicles in each of a number of groups. All injury accident involvements are included, regardless of whether the injured person was inside the car or not. Information is shown by size of car, private or company ownership, age of car, and by severity of injury.

The purpose of Table 1 is to illustrate differences in the rate of involvement in injury accidents of different types, sizes and ages of car. It is important to remember that differences in rate between groups in Table 1 will strongly reflect differences in the level and type of use and of driver behaviour, and should be interpreted carefully. General information on car use, by age of car, engine capacity and ownership, extracted from the National Travel Survey, is summarised in Appendix 1.

Table 3 repeats the rates of involvement as presented in Table 1, but broken down to show results for individual models of car. These are expressed as rates per 10,000 licensed vehicles of each particular model. As emphasised above, there may be considerable differences in the level of use and type of driver. Comparisons between models in different groups could be misleading and are not recommended. Within a group of cars, the differences in usage between models of car are likely to be smaller but will still have a considerable influence on the rates tabulated.

Table 2 shows car user casualty rates per 10,000 licensed vehicles. Only persons injured while travelling inside the car are included in these rates. Information is shown by size of car, private or company ownership, and by severity of injury to occupant.

Table 4 repeats the car user casualty rates depicted in Table 2, but broken down to show results for individual models of car. The comments made above about comparisons between models in Table 3 are equally applicable to Table 4. However the average number of passengers carried has a much greater influence on the rates presented in Tables 2 and 4. The accident reporting system does not require the police to record the number of uninjured passengers, so it is difficult to assess the size of this influence on the figures presented.

Section 2: Risk of injury to drivers involved in injury accidents

Tables 5 and 6 provide information to allow an assessment of the secondary safety records of different types and models of car. They show the percentage of injury accidents involving collision with a vehicle or other hard object which result in injury to the driver. Accidents involving just a single car and pedestrians or two wheeled vehicles are excluded because they pose only a very small risk of injury to the driver. Driver injuries are considered because all cars have a single driver exposed to risk of injury, except parked cars which were excluded from the analysis. The average number of passengers carried does have an influence on the figures presented, but this effect is likely to be small.

The effects of various accident characteristics on the risk of driver injury when involved in an injury accident are shown in Table 5. The percentages are derived using a statistical modelling technique. The most important consequence of analysing the data in this way is that the estimates of injury risk are independent of each other. For example, the estimates of injury risk on different road types are the best available estimates of the specific effect of road type, after the influences of variations in the other effects listed have been removed. In practice, there are interactions between the factors in Table 5, so that for example the effect of type of object hit is not the same on a 30 mph road as on a 70 mph road. The risks shown in the table relate to the average specific effects of those factors in injury accidents. Further explanation and information on the analyses are given in Appendix 2.

Table 6 shows the percentage of car drivers injured when involved in an injury accident for individual models of car. The percentages are derived from statistical models similar to those used for Table 5, but extended to allow for the effect of model of car. This enables fairer comparisons to be made between car models, because the percentages are corrected to allow for differences in the types of accident that cars are involved in. For example, Table 5 reveals that accidents on roads with a higher speed limit are generally more severe than those on other roads. A car model having a high proportion of its accidents on roads of this type would be unfairly assessed if these corrections were not made.

The 1989 report did not make these statistical corrections. For comparison, Table 6 in this report also shows the corresponding uncorrected estimates of injury risk in brackets. It is apparent that the differences between the uncorrected and corrected figures are relatively small.

3.4. Range of groups and models covered

The reliability of each accident involvement and casualty rate presented in Section 1 depends on the number of licensed cars in that category. For this reason, the rates are not quoted for car types or models with populations of less than 20,000 licensed vehicles. Fatality rates are not quoted for individual car models because they cannot be estimated reliably from the small number of fatalities observed.

The data presented in Tables 1 and 2 and also in the summary lines of Tables 3 and 4 include all cars involved in injury accidents and not just those types and models specifically identified because they are above the 20,000 licensed vehicles threshold.

In Table 6, car models are only shown where the statistical analysis indicates that the estimated driver injury percentages are likely to be accurate to within ±2.0 for fatal or serious injuries and ±5.0 for all casualty severities. This is a tighter criterion than that used in the 1989 report. The results for the more common models of car have a higher level of accuracy.

3.5. Other publications

Similar reports on car safety have been published in the United States of America by the Insurance Institute for Highway Safety, and in Sweden by the Folksam Insurance Company. Each produces a summary report for widespread distribution, and an accompanying detailed explanatory booklet describing the methods employed.

The American summary report only deals with deaths to car occupants. It covers a three year period, and reports fatality rates for models with more than 150,000 registrations during that time. Results are grouped by size of car.

The Swedish summary report does not include any details of the methods employed, and classifies cars as safer than average, average, or less safe than average. These assessments are given regardless of the size of car, although supplementary indicators are provided to show those cars safer than average in each weight band.

4. Results

4.1. Table 1: Rates of involvement in injury accidents: by size of car and ownership

Interpretation of the figures in this table depends on the relative mileages of the different types of car, their pattern of use and the behaviour of their drivers.

Each year, drivers of privately owned standard performance cars are involved in between 2 and 3 fatal accidents and between 20 and 30 serious accidents for every 10,000 licensed vehicles. Drivers of similar cars in company ownership are generally involved in greater numbers of accidents. This may be partly explained by The National Travel Survey data which shows that in general company owned cars record higher mileages than privately owned cars.

Drivers of both new and old privately owned high performance cars generally have higher rates of involvement in injury accidents than drivers of their standard performance counterparts. Fatal accident involvement rates of high performance cars are about double their standard performance counterparts and serious accident involvement rates are nearly 50 percent higher. During 1990, small high performance cars registered before 1988 had the worst overall record, with 63 involvements in fatal or serious accidents per 10,000 licensed vehicles.

Newer cars are seen to have lower rates of involvement in injury accidents than older cars, despite the evidence in Appendix 1 which shows that newer cars on average cover more miles each year.

4.2. Table 2: Car user casualty rates: by size of car and ownership

Again, interpretation of the figures in this table depends on the relative mileages of the different types of car, their patterns of use and the behaviour of their drivers.

Each year about one car user is killed and about 10 seriously injured for every 10,000 licensed vehicles. The car user casualty rates show a tendency to decline with increasing size of car, although the relationship is less strong for more serious casualties.

New company and privately owned cars have very similar casualty rates overall. Small and small/medium company owned cars have higher rates of injury than the corresponding privately owned cars, but the reverse is true of large cars. Among older cars, company owned vehicles have generally lower casualty rates than privately owned vehicles. Overall, newer cars have lower casualty rates than older cars. The National Travel Survey evidence is that company cars record higher mileages than privately owned cars, and that newer cars record higher mileages than older cars.

High performance cars generally have higher casualty rates than their standard performance counterparts. This is particularly true of the small car group, for which the high performance vehicles have a much higher rate of injuries, and generally about twice the rate of deaths and serious injuries, as the standard performance vehicles.

4.3. Table 3: Rates of involvement in injury accidents: by make/model and ownership

Table 4: Car user casualty rates: by make/model and ownership

Tables 3 and 4 are based on observations of cars involved in injury accidents during 1990. Future involvement rates are, however, subject to uncertainty. It is emphasised again that accident and casualty rates depend mainly on driver behaviour and on average mileages, among other factors, as well as on the safety design of the car.

The rates are subject to random fluctuations, depending on the number of cars of each model. Those rates marked with an asterisk provide strong evidence that rate for the model and its drivers is genuinely different from the average for the group. An explanation of the statistical tests used is given in Appendix 2.

4.4. Table 5: Risk of injury to drivers involved in injury accidents: by various factors

The rates shown relate to the average specific effects of those factors in injury accidents, after correcting for the influences of variations in the other factors listed. For example, the risks of injury tabulated for different sizes of car are corrected to allow for differences in the age and sex of their drivers.

Of the factors considered, those having the most influence on the risk of death or serious injury when involved in an injury accident are the speed limit of road, the type of object hit and the first point of impact. The most severe accidents occur on 60 mph roads, where the risk of death or serious injury to the driver in an accident is 3 times higher than on a 20 or 30 mph road. The risk of death or serious injury is about one third lower on a 70 mph than on a 60 mph road, which is perhaps a reflection of the improved segregation of traffic on dual carriageway roads.

Age is not a large influence on risk of injury when involved in an accident, although there is an increased susceptibility to death or serious injury in the over 55 age group. Women are less likely to be killed when involved in an accident, which may indicate involvement at lower impact speeds. However, they are about 50 percent more likely to be injured when involved in an accident than men. This is surprising, but could be due to a higher level of injury accident reporting among women, rather than a greater real risk of injury.

A driver of a small car is about 50 percent more likely to be injured when involved in an injury accident than a driver of a large car. The risk of death to a car driver when involved in a collision with a heavy vehicle such as a heavy goods vehicle is more than 5 times the risk of death when involved in a collision with a light vehicle such as a car.

4.5. Table 6: Risk of injury to drivers involved in injury accidents: by make/model

The most striking observation from the data in Table 6 is the similarity in the percentage of drivers injured between car models within a size group. The risk of death or serious injury to the driver involved in an injury accident is about 50 percent higher for the worst models in a group than for the best. The risk of slight injuries shows a smaller variation between car models.

The risks shown for each model of car are subject to random fluctuations, depending on the number of recorded accident involvements. Those rates marked with an asterisk provide strong evidence that rate for the car model is genuinely different from the average for the group.

References:- Insurance Institute for Highway Safety: Status Report. Vol 24, No 11.
1005 North Glebe Road, Arlington, VA 22201. ISSN 0018-988X.

Safe and Dangerous Cars 1989-90: A report from Folksam.
Folksam, Division for Research and Development, S-106 60 Stockholm.

DEFINITIONS

The statistics refer to accidents involving cars resulting in personal injury on public roads, including footways, which became known to the police. Results for 1990 include all accidents in that year determined by the date of accident. Tables in Section 2 also include data from 1989 accidents. Figures for deaths refer to persons who sustained injuries causing death at the time of the accident or within 30 days of the accident, which is the internationally recognised definition.

Injury severity	*Severity* of an *injury* to a casualty is determined by the degree of injury and is either *fatal, seriously injured* or *slightly injured*.
Accident Severity	*Severity* of an *accident*, is determined by the severity of injury of the most severely injured casualty in that accident. That is *fatal*, where one or more persons involved in the accident were killed, *serious*, where one or more persons involved in the accident were seriously injured but no-one killed, or *slight*, where one or more persons involved in the accident were slightly injured but no-one killed or seriously injured.
Car	Any four-wheeled car. This includes saloons, hatch-backs, estates, "people carriers", coupes and convertibles. Purpose-built taxis, car derived vans, goods vehicles and minibuses are not included.
Size	Not formally defined but arranged so that the consumer can recognise standard groups. As an approximate guide, cars in the *small* group are generally between 140 and 150 inches in length, those in the *small/medium* group between 155 and 165 inches, those in the *medium* group between 170 and 180 inches, and those in the *large* group over 180 inches.
	The allocation of a particular model to a size group does not imply that the model meets any formal classification or standard.
High performance	No single criterion has been adopted for the purpose of identifying cars in this category. Models whose performance is considerably higher than the standard production range are included. Most will be fitted with engines of higher capacity than their standard performance counterparts, and may also have features such as fuel injection or be fitted with turbo chargers. Typically, though not invariably, they have the capability of accelerating from 0 to 60 mph in 10 seconds or less.
	In the large group most cars are fitted with engines of greater power and higher cubic capacity. There is less distinction between standard and higher performance cars, so all cars in this size group have been classed as standard performance.
New and *Old* cars	Used in this report to describe cars registered on or after 1st January 1988 and before 1st January 1988 respectively. That is *new*, to describe cars up to three years old at the end of 1990, and *old*, to describe cars three years old or more at the same date.
Ownership type	Identified from the registered keeper record at DVLA. *Company* cars are registered in the name of a company or partnership. *Private* cars are registered in the name of an individual.

Table 1: Rates of involvement in injury accidents: by size of car and ownership: 1990

Injury accident involvements per 10,000 licensed vehicles in each group

Age of car / Performance / Size	Privately owned				Company owned		
	Injury accident severity				Injury accident severity		
	Fatal	Serious	All		Fatal	Serious	All
Regd. on or since 1.1.88							
Standard							
Small	1.6	21	123		2.4	29	178
Small/medium	2.2	22	127		3.5	31	199
Medium	2.5	24	132		3.4	27	163
Large	2.4	21	110		3.1	22	123
All standard	2.1	22	125		3.2	27	166
High							
Small	5.5	34	182		3.6	36	196
Small/medium	4.3	32	168		3.3	29	176
Medium	5.1	29	135		4.1	28	142
All high	4.8	32	163		3.7	30	162
Registered before 1.1.88							
Standard							
Small	2.4	27	159		2.2	26	148
Small/medium	2.8	32	178		4.0	39	226
Medium	3.1	34	187		3.7	37	218
Large	2.8	27	148		2.9	23	139
All standard	2.8	31	172		3.1	32	186
High							
Small	6.1	57	284		..	..	..
Small/medium	5.3	45	230		..	..	..
Medium	4.9	38	195		..	..	..
All high	5.3	45	228		5.0	39	209

Notes

.. Denotes fewer than 20,000 licensed vehicles in the group.

Table 2: Car user casualty rates: by size of car and ownership: 1990

	Car user casualties per 10,000 licensed vehicles in each group						
Age of car	Privately owned				Company owned		
Performance	Injury severity				Injury severity		
Size	Fatal	Serious	All		Fatal	Serious	All
Regd. on or since 1.1.88							
Standard							
Small	0.8	11	85		1.0	15	112
Small/medium	1.2	11	79		1.3	14	101
Medium	0.9	11	75		1.0	10	76
Large	0.9	9	52		0.8	7	47
All standard	1.0	11	78		1.0	11	81
High							
Small	2.9	19	127		3.1	16	117
Small/medium	2.0	18	100		0.6	11	89
Medium	2.7	17	82		1.4	13	68
All high	2.4	18	102		1.3	13	83
Registered before 1.1.88							
Standard							
Small	1.4	16	115		0.6	14	100
Small/medium	1.4	17	117		1.9	18	126
Medium	1.3	15	107		1.3	14	108
Large	0.9	10	68		0.8	7	54
All standard	1.3	15	109		1.2	13	97
High							
Small	2.9	37	201		..	..	..
Small/medium	3.2	24	144		..	..	..
Medium	1.9	16	109		..	..	..
All high	2.9	23	142		2.5	17	122

Notes

.. Denotes fewer than 20,000 licensed vehicles in the group.

Table 3: Rates of involvement in injury accidents: by make/model and ownership: 1990

Injury accident involvements per 10,000 licensed vehicles of each model

Age of car Performance Size/Model[1]		Privately owned Injury accident severity		Company owned Injury accident severity	
		Fatal or Serious	All	Fatal or Serious	All
Registered on or since 1.1.88					
Standard					
Small					
CITROEN	AX	24	117	..	..
FIAT	PANDA	25	137	..	..
FIAT	UNO	29 *	153 *	..	..
FORD	FIESTA	25	132 *	32	200 *
NISSAN	MICRA	19	112 *	..	..
PEUGEOT	205	23	116	29	157
RENAULT	5	22	121	..	..
ROVER	METRO	22	117	31	160
ROVER	MINI	27	137	..	..
VAUXHALL	NOVA	22	123	37	205
VOLKSWAGEN	POLO	17 *	105 *	..	..
ALL SMALL[2]		23	123	31	178
Small/medium					
FIAT	TIPO	23	123	..	..
FORD	ESCORT	28 *	145 *	37	242 *
FORD	ORION	30 *	161 *	35	209
HONDA	CIVIC	18	90 *	..	..
LADA	RIVA	28	130	..	..
LADA	SAMARA	25	131	..	..
MAZDA	323	15 *	86 *	..	..
NISSAN	SUNNY	22	122	..	..
PEUGEOT	309	24	115	35	204
RENAULT	19	22	94 *	..	..
ROVER	200 SERIES	24	112 *	33	161 *
ROVER	MAESTRO	22	118	38	206
TOYOTA	COROLLA	18 *	99 *	..	..
VAUXHALL	ASTRA	28	142 *	34	197
VAUXHALL	BELMONT	22	129	..	..
VOLKSWAGEN	GOLF	19 *	104 *	27	160 *
ALL SMALL/MEDIUM[2]		24	127	34	199
Medium					
BMW	3 SERIES	25	121	20 *	137 *
CITROEN	BX	27	137	37	187 *
FORD	SAPPHIRE	32	162 *	37 *	192 *
FORD	SIERRA	31	152 *	34	184 *
PEUGEOT	405	31	159 *	33	164
ROVER	MONTEGO	30	144	34	173
TOYOTA	CARINA	24	106 *	..	..
VAUXHALL	CAVALIER	30	141	30	156
VOLVO	340	21 *	97 *	..	..
ALL MEDIUM[2]		26	132	30	163
Large					
BMW	5 SERIES	..	..	22	109
FORD	GRANADA	34	135 *	26	132
ROVER	800 SERIES	30	134 *	32	150 *
VAUXHALL	CARLTON	31	130	25	134
VOLVO	740	17	108	26	121
ALL LARGE[2]		23	110	25	123

Notes

1 Models are listed under the current market name of the manufacturer.
2 Includes models not specifically identified.
* Indicates that the difference between the rate for the model and its associated drivers and the group average has at most a 1% possibility of arising by chance. See text.
.. Denotes fewer than 20,000 licensed vehicles in the group.

Table 3 (cont.): Rates of involvement in injury accidents: by make/model and ownership: 1990

Injury accident involvements per 10,000 licensed vehicles of each model

Age of car Performance Size/Model[1]		Privately owned		Company owned	
		Injury accident severity		Injury accident severity	
		Fatal or Serious	All	Fatal or Serious	All
Registered before 1.1.88					
Standard					
Small					
CITROEN	2CV	19 *	121 *	..	..
CITROEN	VISA	27	154	..	..
FIAT	127	46 *	209 *	..	..
FIAT	PANDA	29	166	..	..
FIAT	UNO	26	154	..	..
FORD	FIESTA	31	169 *	30	158
NISSAN	CHERRY	33	179 *	..	..
NISSAN	MICRA	25 *	139 *	..	..
PEUGEOT	205	29	141 *	..	..
PEUGEOT	SAMBA	24	148	..	..
PEUGEOT	SUNBEAM	47 *	206 *	..	..
RENAULT	5	34	166	..	..
ROVER	METRO	26 *	144 *	22	122 *
ROVER	MINI	33 *	175 *	..	..
TOYOTA	STARLET	33	162	..	..
VAUXHALL	NOVA	28	150 *	..	..
VOLKSWAGEN	BEETLE	28	159	..	..
VOLKSWAGEN	POLO	26 *	139 *	..	..
ALL SMALL[2]		29	159	28	148
Small/medium					
FIAT	REGATA	33	175	..	..
FIAT	STRADA	50 *	221 *	..	..
FORD	ESCORT	41 *	214 *	47	255 *
FORD	ORION	36	193 *	..	..
HONDA	CIVIC	28	148 *	..	..
LADA	RIVA	27 *	128 *	..	..
MAZDA	323	24 *	141 *	..	..
NISSAN	SUNNY	34	181	..	..
PEUGEOT	305	36	156 *	..	..
PEUGEOT	309	31	149 *	..	..
PEUGEOT	AVENGER	34	190	..	..
PEUGEOT	HORIZON	26 *	156 *	..	..
RENAULT	11	26 *	150 *	..	..
RENAULT	9	27 *	158 *	..	..
ROVER	1100	41	216 *	..	..
ROVER	200 SERIES	23 *	129 *	..	..
ROVER	ACCLAIM	31	149 *	..	..
ROVER	ALLEGRO	25 *	138 *	..	..
ROVER	DOLOMITE	34	165	..	..
ROVER	MAESTRO	27 *	135 *	..	..
SKODA	ESTELLE 2	23 *	133 *	..	..
TOYOTA	COROLLA	30	170	..	..
VAUXHALL	ASTRA	34	172	44	283 *
VAUXHALL	BELMONT	32	158	..	..
VAUXHALL	CHEVETTE	36	183	..	..
VAUXHALL	KADETT	42	209 *	..	..
VAUXHALL	VIVA	35	190	..	..
VOLKSWAGEN	GOLF	31 *	155 *	..	..
ALL SMALL/MEDIUM[2]		35	178	43	226

Notes

1 Models are listed under the current market name of the manufacturer.
2 Includes models not specifically identified.
* Indicates that the difference between the rate for the model and its associated drivers and the group average has at most a 1% possibility of arising by chance. See text.
.. Denotes fewer than 20,000 licensed vehicles in the group.

Table 3 (cont.): Rates of involvement in injury accidents: by make/model and ownership: 1990

Injury accident involvements per 10,000 licensed vehicles of each model

Age of car Performance Size/Model[1]		Privately owned Injury accident severity		Company owned Injury accident severity	
		Fatal or Serious	All	Fatal or Serious	All
Registered before 1.1.88					
Standard					
Medium					
AUDI	80	32	175	..	..
BMW	3 SERIES	42	188	..	..
CITROEN	BX	30	157 *	..	..
FORD	CAPRI	54 *	258 *	..	..
FORD	CORTINA	47 *	243 *	..	..
FORD	SAPPHIRE	34	172	..	..
FORD	SIERRA	33 *	184	50	257 *
MAZDA	626	38	165 *	..	..
NISSAN	BLUEBIRD	47 *	253 *	..	..
NISSAN	STANZA	31	183	..	..
PEUGEOT	ALPINE	40	180	..	..
PEUGEOT	SOLARA	36	155 *	..	..
RENAULT	18	34	181	..	..
ROVER	AMBASSADOR[3]	31 *	151 *	..	..
ROVER	ITAL	30 *	160 *	..	..
ROVER	MARINA	39	191	..	..
ROVER	MAXI	26 *	134 *	..	..
ROVER	MONTEGO	32 *	167 *	..	..
TOYOTA	CARINA	34	176	..	..
TOYOTA	CELICA	45	234 *	..	..
VAUXHALL	CAVALIER	37	186	49	251 *
VAUXHALL	MANTA	47	230 *	..	..
VOLKSWAGEN	JETTA	34	156 *	..	..
VOLKSWAGEN	PASSAT	29 *	139 *	..	..
VOLVO	340	20 *	107 *	..	..
VOLVO	343	25 *	140 *	..	..
VOLVO	345	23 *	132 *	..	..
VOLVO	360	25 *	124 *	..	..
ALL MEDIUM[2]		37	187	41	218
Large					
AUDI	100	33	188 *	..	..
BMW	5 SERIES	41 *	171 *	..	..
FORD	GRANADA	37 *	182 *	41 *	209 *
HONDA	ACCORD	29	171 *	..	..
MERCEDES	W123/4 SALOON	22 *	141	..	..
PEUGEOT	505	38	164	..	..
RENAULT	25	26	162	..	..
ROVER	2000	41	138	..	..
ROVER	2600	42 *	183 *	..	..
ROVER	3500	46 *	195 *	..	..
ROVER	RANGEROVER	21 *	109 *	..	..
SAAB	900	33	141	..	..
VAUXHALL	CARLTON	27	150	..	..
VOLVO	240	25	111 *	..	..
VOLVO	244	24	134	..	..
VOLVO	245	25	124 *	..	..
VOLVO	740	27	134	..	..
ALL LARGE[2]		30	148	26	139

Notes

1 Models are listed under the current market name of the manufacturer.
2 Includes models not specifically identified.
3 Includes Princess models.
* Indicates that the difference between the rate for the model and its associated drivers and the group average has at most a 1% possibility of arising by chance. See text.
.. Denotes fewer than 20,000 licensed vehicles in the group.

13

Table 4: Car user casualty rates: by make/model and ownership: 1990

Car user casualties per 10,000 licensed vehicles of each model

Age of car Performance Size/Model[1]	Privately owned Injury severity Fatal or Serious	All	Company owned Injury severity Fatal or Serious	All
Registered on or since 1.1.88				
Standard				
Small				
CITROEN AX	14	83	..	..
FIAT PANDA	14	94	..	..
FIAT UNO	18 *	104 *	..	..
FORD FIESTA	12	93 *	16	125 *
NISSAN MICRA	11	75 *	..	..
PEUGEOT 205	13	75 *	10	100
RENAULT 5	12	86	..	..
ROVER METRO	11	81	16	101
ROVER MINI	17	104 *	..	..
VAUXHALL NOVA	11	84	18	119
VOLKSWAGEN POLO	8 *	67 *	..	..
ALL SMALL[2]	12	85	16	112
Small/medium				
FIAT TIPO	11	74	..	..
FORD ESCORT	14 *	95 *	16	129 *
FORD ORION	16 *	104 *	15	101
HONDA CIVIC	5 *	52 *	..	..
LADA RIVA	8	62 *	..	..
LADA SAMARA	12	83	..	..
MAZDA 323	6 *	46 *	..	..
NISSAN SUNNY	9	72	..	..
PEUGEOT 309	15	80	14	113
RENAULT 19	10	57 *	..	..
ROVER 200 SERIES	12	72	15	81 *
ROVER MAESTRO	11	72	18	100
TOYOTA COROLLA	8 *	49 *	..	..
VAUXHALL ASTRA	13	87 *	14	95
VAUXHALL BELMONT	7 *	75	..	..
VOLKSWAGEN GOLF	8 *	58 *	12	77 *
ALL SMALL/MEDIUM[2]	12	79	15	101
Medium				
BMW 3 SERIES	9	66	8	64
CITROEN BX	10	69	12	74
FORD SAPPHIRE	16	103 *	12	93 *
FORD SIERRA	17 *	95 *	13	88 *
PEUGEOT 405	12	86	10	70
ROVER MONTEGO	13	82	11	87 *
TOYOTA CARINA	13	59	..	..
VAUXHALL CAVALIER	13	77	10	72
VOLVO 340	10	59 *	..	..
ALL MEDIUM[2]	12	75	11	76
Large				
BMW 5 SERIES	..	..	5	35 *
FORD GRANADA	14	75 *	10	54
ROVER 800 SERIES	14	66	10	53
VAUXHALL CARLTON	15	68	8	53
VOLVO 740	10	47	4 *	36 *
ALL LARGE[2]	10	52	8	47

Notes

1 Models are listed under the current market name of the manufacturer.
2 Includes models not specifically identified.
* Indicates that the difference between the rate for the model and its associated drivers and the group average has at most a 1% possibility of arising by chance. See text.
.. Denotes fewer than 20,000 licensed vehicles in the group.

Table 4 (cont.): Car user casualty rates: by make/model and ownership: 1990

	Car user casualties per 10,000 licensed vehicles of each model			
Age of car	Privately owned		Company owned	
Performance	Injury severity		Injury severity	
Size/Model[1]	Fatal or Serious	All	Fatal or Serious	All

Registered before 1.1.88

Standard

Small

CITROEN	2CV	13		94	*	..	..
CITROEN	VISA	18		119		..	..
FIAT	127	29	*	149	*	..	..
FIAT	PANDA	16		116		..	..
FIAT	UNO	15		101	*	..	..
FORD	FIESTA	16		116		13	97
NISSAN	CHERRY	17		117		..	..
NISSAN	MICRA	11	*	91	*	..	..
PEUGEOT	205	16		97	*	..	..
PEUGEOT	SAMBA	11	*	107		..	..
PEUGEOT	SUNBEAM	34	*	150	*	..	..
RENAULT	5	20		118		..	..
ROVER	METRO	16		109	*	13	100
ROVER	MINI	23	*	144	*	..	..
TOYOTA	STARLET	14		106		..	..
VAUXHALL	NOVA	14	*	101	*	..	..
VOLKSWAGEN	BEETLE	13		107		..	..
VOLKSWAGEN	POLO	14	*	96	*	..	..
ALL SMALL[2]		17		115		15	100

Small/medium

FIAT	REGATA	15		104		..	..
FIAT	STRADA	28	*	148	*	..	..
FORD	ESCORT	24	*	149	*	23	149 *
FORD	ORION	17		123		..	..
HONDA	CIVIC	15		93	*	..	..
LADA	RIVA	11	*	80	*	..	..
MAZDA	323	12	*	90	*	..	..
NISSAN	SUNNY	17		110	*	..	..
PEUGEOT	305	19		89	*	..	..
PEUGEOT	309	16		109		..	..
PEUGEOT	AVENGER	18		116		..	..
PEUGEOT	HORIZON	14		104	*	..	..
RENAULT	11	12	*	91	*	..	..
RENAULT	9	12	*	101	*	..	..
ROVER	1100	26		170	*	..	..
ROVER	200 SERIES	12	*	77	*	..	..
ROVER	ACCLAIM	16		102	*	..	..
ROVER	ALLEGRO	14	*	95	*	..	..
ROVER	DOLOMITE	16		102		..	..
ROVER	MAESTRO	14	*	88	*	..	..
SKODA	ESTELLE 2	10	*	94	*	..	..
TOYOTA	COROLLA	14	*	97	*	..	..
VAUXHALL	ASTRA	15	*	103	*	16	145
VAUXHALL	BELMONT	17		106		..	..
VAUXHALL	CHEVETTE	20		128	*	..	..
VAUXHALL	KADETT	24		146	*	..	..
VAUXHALL	VIVA	18		126		..	..
VOLKSWAGEN	GOLF	14	*	96	*	..	..
ALL SMALL/MEDIUM[2]		18		117		20	126

Notes

1 Models are listed under the current market name of the manufacturer.
2 Includes models not specifically identified.
* Indicates that the difference between the rate for the model and its associated drivers and the group average has at most a 1% possibility of arising by chance. See text.
.. Denotes fewer than 20,000 licensed vehicles in the group.

Table 4 (cont.): Car user casualty rates: by make/model and ownership: 1990

Car user casualties per 10,000 licensed vehicles of each model

Age of car		Privately owned		Company owned	
Performance		Injury severity		Injury severity	
Size/Model[1]		Fatal or Serious	All	Fatal or Serious	All
Registered before 1.1.88					
Standard					
Medium					
AUDI	80	16	107	..	..
BMW	3 SERIES	21 *	101	..	..
CITROEN	BX	14	86 *	..	..
FORD	CAPRI	27 *	153 *	..	..
FORD	CORTINA	23 *	144 *	..	..
FORD	SAPPHIRE	12	93	..	..
FORD	SIERRA	13 *	102 *	19	123
MAZDA	626	14	83 *	..	..
NISSAN	BLUEBIRD	18	133 *	..	..
NISSAN	STANZA	18	116	..	..
PEUGEOT	ALPINE	16	109	..	..
PEUGEOT	SOLARA	15	85 *	..	..
RENAULT	18	16	108	..	..
ROVER	AMBASSADOR[3]	12 *	77 *	..	..
ROVER	ITAL	17	103	..	..
ROVER	MARINA	22 *	134 *	..	..
ROVER	MAXI	14	79 *	..	..
ROVER	MONTEGO	14	96 *	..	..
TOYOTA	CARINA	18	103	..	..
TOYOTA	CELICA	16	122	..	..
VAUXHALL	CAVALIER	15 *	105	15	125
VAUXHALL	MANTA	20	136 *	..	..
VOLKSWAGEN	JETTA	14	94	..	..
VOLKSWAGEN	PASSAT	12 *	75 *	..	..
VOLVO	340	10 *	63 *	..	..
VOLVO	343	10 *	83 *	..	..
VOLVO	345	10 *	72 *	..	..
VOLVO	360	11 *	61 *	..	..
ALL MEDIUM[2]		16	107	15	108
Large					
AUDI	100	9	82	..	..
BMW	5 SERIES	18 *	89 *	..	..
FORD	GRANADA	14 *	86 *	11	97 *
HONDA	ACCORD	16 *	94 *	..	..
MERCEDES	W123/4 SALOON	7	57	..	..
PEUGEOT	505	18	93 *	..	..
RENAULT	25	5 *	63	..	..
ROVER	2000	12	64	..	..
ROVER	2600	20 *	99 *	..	..
ROVER	3500	18	100 *	..	..
ROVER	RANGEROVER	6 *	36 *	..	..
SAAB	900	11	69	..	..
VAUXHALL	CARLTON	7 *	71	..	..
VOLVO	240	7 *	44 *	..	..
VOLVO	244	6 *	57 *	..	..
VOLVO	245	9	54 *	..	..
VOLVO	740	7	51 *	..	..
ALL LARGE[2]		11	68	8	54

Notes

1 Models are listed under the current market name of the manufacturer.
2 Includes models not specifically identified.
3 Includes Princess models.
* Indicates that the difference between the rate for the model and its associated drivers and the group average has at most a 1% possibility of arising by chance. See text.
.. Denotes fewer than 20,000 licensed vehicles in the group.

Table 5: Risk of injury to drivers involved in injury accidents: by various factors: 1989 to 1990

Percentage of drivers injured when involved in an injury accident[1]

Performance Factor	Injury severity[2]		
	Fatal	Fatal or Serious	All
Standard			
Type of object hit			
Light vehicle[3]	0.6	7	47
Heavy vehicle[4]	3.3	17	74
Other hard object	1.2	13	73
Speed limit of road (mph)			
20 or 30	0.3	5	49
40 or 50	0.8	8	52
60	2.3	15	60
70	1.8	10	50
Sex of driver			
Male	0.8	8	45
Female	0.5	9	67
Age of driver			
17 - 24	0.7	8	54
25 - 34	0.6	8	52
35 - 54	0.7	8	51
55 or more	1.3	11	55
Size of car			
Small	0.9	9	60
Small/medium	0.7	8	53
Medium	0.6	7	49
Large	0.6	6	41
First point of impact			
Front	0.9	11	51
Back	0.2	3	54
Offside	1.6	11	60
Nearside	1.0	8	50
All accidents	0.7	8	53

Notes

1 Excluding accidents involving just a single car and pedestrians or two-wheeled vehicles.
2 Corrected for influences of variations in the other factors listed.
3 Cars, minibuses, light goods vehicles, etc.
4 Heavy goods vehicles, buses, coaches, etc.

Table 6: Risk of injury to drivers involved in injury accidents: by size of car and make/model: 1989 to 1990

Percentage of drivers injured when involved in an injury accident[1]

Performance			Injury severity[2]			
Size/Model[3]		Registration dates	Fatal or Serious		All	
Standard						
Small						
FIAT	PANDA	Jun 81[4] - Dec 90	10	(9)	60	(64)
FIAT	UNO	Jun 83[4] - Jan 90	11	(10)	60	(61)
FORD	FIESTA	Jan 81 - Mar 89	9	(9)	60	(62)
FORD	FIESTA	Apr 89 - Dec 90[5]	8	(8)	58	(58)
NISSAN	CHERRY	Sep 82 - Aug 86[5]	9	(8)	56	(55)
NISSAN	MICRA	Jun 83[4] - Dec 90	10	(9)	59	(60)
PEUGEOT	205	Oct 83[4] - Dec 90	9	(10)	57 *	(59)
RENAULT	5	Jan 81 - Jan 85	9	(10)	58	(62)
RENAULT	5	Feb 85 - Dec 90	10	(10)	61	(63)
ROVER	METRO	Jan 81 - Apr 90	9	(9)	61	(64)
ROVER	MINI	Jan 81 - Dec 90	12 *	(12)	67 *	(71)
VAUXHALL	NOVA	Apr 83[4] - Dec 90	9	(8)	58	(60)
VOLKSWAGEN	POLO	Feb 82 - Oct 90	9	(9)	59	(61)
ALL SMALL[6]		Jan 81 - Dec 90	9	(9)	60	(62)
Small/medium						
FORD	ESCORT	Jan 81 - Aug 90	9	(8)	55 *	(54)
FORD	ORION	Sep 83[4] - Aug 90	8	(8)	54	(51)
LADA	RIVA[7]	Jan 81 - Dec 90	8	(8)	53	(49)
NISSAN	SUNNY	May 82 - Aug 86	8	(7)	56	(52)
NISSAN	SUNNY	Sep 86 - Dec 90	9	(8)	50	(48)
PEUGEOT	309	Feb 86[4] - Dec 90[5]	9	(9)	55	(55)
RENAULT	11	Jul 83[4] - Feb 89[5]	9	(9)	53	(53)
ROVER	200 SERIES	Jun 84[4] - Sep 89	8	(8)	51	(48)
ROVER	ACCLAIM	Oct 81[4] - Jun 84[5]	9	(9)	55	(54)
ROVER	MAESTRO	Mar 83[4] - Dec 90	8	(8)	50 *	(48)
VAUXHALL	ASTRA[8]	Jan 81 - Sep 84	7	(7)	52	(50)
VAUXHALL	ASTRA	Oct 84 - Dec 90	8	(8)	52	(50)
VAUXHALL	BELMONT	Jan 86[4] - Dec 90[5]	6	(6)	50	(45)
VAUXHALL	CHEVETTE	Jan 81 - Aug 84[5]	9	(9)	55	(55)
VOLKSWAGEN	GOLF	May 84 - Dec 90	6 *	(6)	49 *	(49)
ALL SMALL/MEDIUM[6]		Jan 81 - Dec 90	8	(8)	53	(52)
Medium						
BMW	3 SERIES	Mar 83 - Dec 90	9	(8)	49	(46)
CITROEN	BX	Aug 83[4] - Dec 90[5]	7	(7)	46	(42)
FORD	CAPRI	Jan 81 - Mar 87[5]	9	(8)	50	(46)
FORD	CORTINA	Jan 81 - Sep 82[5]	8	(7)	51	(47)
FORD	SAPPHIRE	Mar 87[4] - Dec 90	7	(7)	51	(47)
FORD	SIERRA	Oct 82[4] - Dec 90[5]	7	(7)	50	(46)
NISSAN	BLUEBIRD	Mar 86 - Sep 90[5]	7	(6)	48	(42)
PEUGEOT	405	Jan 88[4] - Dec 90[5]	7	(7)	46	(42)
RENAULT	18	Jan 81 - May 86[5]	8	(8)	49	(47)
RENAULT	21	Jun 86[4] - Dec 90	7	(7)	43 *	(40)
ROVER	MONTEGO	Apr 84[4] - Dec 90	8	(8)	48	(44)
VAUXHALL	CAVALIER	Aug 81 - Sep 88	7	(6)	49	(45)
VAUXHALL	CAVALIER	Oct 88 - Dec 90	7	(7)	46	(41)
VOLVO	300 SERIES	Jan 81 - Dec 90	7	(8)	48	(48)
ALL MEDIUM[6]		Jan 81 - Dec 90	7	(7)	49	(45)

Notes

1 Excluding accidents involving just a single car and pedestrians or two-wheeled vehicles.
2 Corrected for selected accident circumstances. Uncorrected rates shown in brackets. See text.
3 Models are listed under the current market name of the manufacturer.
4 Approximate introduction date. All cars registered from January 1981 are included.
5 Approximate withdrawal date. All cars registered up to December 1990 are included.
6 Includes models not specifically identified.
7 Includes earlier 1200, 1300, 1500 and 1600 models.
8 Includes equivalent Opel Kadett models.
* Indicates that the difference between the rate for the model and the group average has at most a 1% possibility of arising by chance. See text.

Table 6 (cont.): Risk of injury to drivers involved in injury accidents: by size of car and make/model: 1989 to 1990

			Percentage of drivers injured when involved in an injury accident[1]			
Performance			**Injury severity[2]**			
Size/Model[3]		Registration dates	Fatal or Serious		All	
Standard						
Large						
AUDI	100/200	Oct 82 - Dec 90	4	(4)	42	(38)
FORD	GRANADA	Jan 81 - Apr 85	7	(5)	42	(35)
FORD	GRANADA	May 85 - Dec 90	7	(7)	45 *	(41)
ROVER	800 SERIES	Jul 86[4] - Dec 90	7	(7)	37	(32)
ROVER	SD1	Jan 81 - Nov 86[5]	7	(7)	44	(39)
SAAB	900	Jan 81 - Dec 90	6	(7)	45	(43)
VAUXHALL	CARLTON	Nov 86 - Dec 90	7	(7)	44	(38)
VOLVO	200 SERIES	Jan 81 - Dec 90	6	(6)	39	(36)
VOLVO	700 SERIES	Jul 82[4] - Dec 90	5	(5)	38	(34)
ALL LARGE[6]		Jan 81 - Dec 90	6	(6)	41	(37)

Notes

1 Excluding accidents involving just a single car and pedestrians or two-wheeled vehicles.
2 Corrected for selected accident circumstances. Uncorrected rates shown in brackets. See text.
3 Models are listed under the current market name of the manufacturer.
4 Approximate introduction date. All cars registered from January 1981 are included.
5 Approximate withdrawal date. All cars registered up to December 1990 are included.
6 Includes models not specifically identified.
* Indicates that the difference between the rate for the model and the group average has at most a 1% possibility of arising by chance. See text.

Appendix 1: Information on average mileage drawn from the National Travel Survey 1985/6

1. Estimated annual average mileage for four wheeled cars: by engine capacity

Up to 700cc	701 to 1000 cc	1001 to 1300 cc	1301 to 1500 cc	1501 to 1800 cc	1801 to 2000 cc	2001 to 2500 cc	2501 to 3000 cc	3001 and over	All
5,900	6,600	7,900	8,200	10,400	10,700	12,200	10,900	9,400	8,900

2. Estimated annual average mileage for four wheeled cars: by ownership

Private	Company	All
7,800	17,800	8,900

3. Estimated annual average mileage for four wheeled cars: by age of car

Up to three years

Up to 6 months	6 months to 1.0 year	1.0 years to 1.5 years	1.5 years to 2.0 years	2.0 years to 3.0 years
13,600	13,900	12,600	12,200	10,600

Above three years old

3 years to 4 years	4 years to 5 years	5 years to 6 years	6 years to 7 years	7 years to 8 years	8 years to 10 years	10 years to 13 years	13 years to 18 years	Over 18 years
9,400	8,800	8,500	8,000	7,700	6,900	6,200	4,900	4,200

4. Estimated annual average mileage for four wheeled cars: by age of main driver

17 years	18 years	19 years	20 years	21-25 years	26-29 years	30-39 years	40-49 years
5,400	7,900	7,500	8,900	9,400	9,800	9,900	10,100

50-59 years	60-64 years	65-69 years	70-74 years	75-79 years	80-84 years	85 or more	All
9,000	7,000	5,600	4,500	4,000	3,300	2,000	8,900

Appendix 2: Explanatory notes to statistical analyses

Section 1: Outline of statistical tests used in Tables 3 and 4

In performing the tests of significance shown in Tables 3 and 4 it has been assumed that the risk of an individual driver being involved in an injury accident is such that the number of accident involvements follows a Poisson distribution. This is appropriate since the average risk per year of involvement in an injury accident is very small. In broad terms this means that in each year there is a high probability of no involvement, a low probability of one involvement, and a very low probability of more than one.

The risk of being involved in an accident naturally varies from driver to driver, but on the assumption that the risk for a driver is largely independent of other drivers' risks, the overall rate for a model of car will also follow a Poisson distribution.

With the lower limit of 20,000 cars for each car model assessed, the Poisson distribution for the model can be satisfactorily approximated by a normal distribution with mean equal to its variance. Simple statistical tests have been made to see whether the rates for specific car models and their drivers are likely to be genuinely different from the group average. Allowance was made for the incomplete coverage of accidents, the variance of the estimated rate for the model and the variance of the group mean.

The same analyses were made for Table 4 as for Table 3, though the Poisson distribution may be less appropriate here as a single accident may result in more than one injury.

Where the difference in rate proved significant at the 1 percent probability level, an indicator in the form of an asterisk (*) has been marked alongside the relevant rate. In such cases there is strong evidence that the rate is genuinely different from the mean for the group.

The more cars there are of a particular model, the greater the confidence in the reliability of the result. Cars which are present in large numbers can therefore be judged significantly different from the group average in some instances where they are closer to the group mean than other less common types. An illustration of the procedure for two hypothetical models of car is given below in an example.

Observed results which fail to achieve significance still provide an indication of the underlying accident or casualty rate for the model and its associated drivers. The reliability of each rate depends on the number of cars of the relevant model. For models with only 20,000 licensed cars, 95 percent confidence intervals for the rates in Table 3 would be typically ±8 for the fatal or serious rate and ±19 for the all severities rate. On a similar basis, 95 percent confidence intervals for the rates in Table 4 would be ±6 for the fatal or serious rate and ±15 for the all severities rate.

Appendix 2: Explanatory notes to statistical analyses (cont.)

Illustrative example

Fatal or serious injury (FSI) accident rate

	Model A	Model B
No. of licensed cars (thousands)	80	320
Estimated coverage	80%	80%
No. of cars monitored (thousands)	64	256
Observed FSI accidents	175	700
Observed FSI rate per 10,000 cars	27.34	27.34
Average FSI rate per 10,000 cars in the group	23.30	23.30
Difference between FSI rate and average for the group	4.04	4.04
Variance of FSI rate per 10,000 cars	$175/(6.4)^2$ $=4.27$	$700/(25.6)^2$ $=1.07$
Variance of average FSI rate per 10,000 cars in the group	0.30	0.30
Variance of difference	4.57	1.36
Standard Error (SE) of difference	2.14	1.17
Normal test statistic	$4.04/2.14$ $=1.89$	$4.04/1.17$ $=3.46$
Assessment	Not significant Unlabelled	Significant Labelled *

A significance label is applied in cases where the test statistic is greater than 2.57.

Appendix 2: Explanatory notes to statistical analyses (cont.)

Section 2: Outline of statistical modelling used in Tables 5 and 6

The risk of injury to a driver involved in an accident clearly depends on a range of factors. A low speed accident in a built-up area involving a collision between a car and a pedestrian poses only a very small risk of injury to the car driver. A high speed accident involving a head-on collision between a car and a heavy goods vehicle poses a very high risk of injury to the car driver.

Valid comparisons of the inherent secondary safety records of different models of car are therefore complicated. Involvement in a high proportion of accidents with a low risk of driver injury will tend to produce a better apparent safety record whereas involvement in a high proportion of accidents with a high risk of driver injury will tend to produce a worse apparent safety record.

In order to isolate individual influences, statistical modelling has been used, which works by imagining that the risk of injury depends on a range of factors. The models look at the influences on the logarithm of the odds of injury, sometimes called the logit function, rather than directly at the influences on the proportion of accidents resulting in injury. This technique, known as logistic regression or logistic analysis, allows the influences on the risk of injury to be isolated and treated in an additive way. Unfortunately, the resulting factors are difficult to interpret by a non-specialist readership, so they have therefore been used to calculate corrected estimates of the percentage of drivers injured.

The statistical analyses used for Table 5 form the basis for the make/model comparisons in Table 6. The largest influences on risk of injury to the driver in an accident identified from the statistical models used for Table 5, as well as those showing the greatest variation between car models, are also included in the statistical analyses comparing models of car used for Table 6. A number of interaction effects are also considered. The results are the best available estimates of the underlying secondary safety record, corrected for differences in key accident circumstances that influence the risk of injury to the driver.

The reliability of the result for a model of car in table 6 depends on the number of recorded accident involvements of that model. Individual models of car are only included in Table 6 if the 95 percent confidence limits for the fatal or serious injury rates are ±2.0 or less. 95 percent confidence intervals for the all injury severities rates are ±5.0 or less. This means that less reliable statistics are excluded from Table 6.

The significance of the difference between the risk tabulated for each model and the group mean has been tested statistically. Those risk estimates marked with an asterisk (*) proved significant at the 1 percent probability level. In such cases there is strong evidence that the risk is genuinely different from the mean for the group.

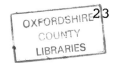

Appendix 2: Explanatory notes to statistical analyses (cont.)

Statistical models used for each injury severity risk in Table 5: –

$$Y_{ijklmn} = \mu + A_i + B_j + C_k + D_l + E_m + F_n + e_{ijklmn},$$

where $Y_{ijklmn} = Log_e [P_{ijklmn}/(1-P_{ijklmn})]$

and $P_{ijklmn} = n_{ijklmn}/N_{ijklmn},$

where N_{ijklmn} = Number of drivers in group $_{ijklmn}$

and n_{ijklmn} = Number of injured drivers in group $_{ijklmn},$

and where the effects are represented by: –

μ	Overall mean,
A_i	Size of car,
B_j	Type of object hit,
C_k	Speed limit of road,
D_l	First point of impact,
E_m	Sex of driver,
F_n	Age group of driver, and
e	Error term.

Statistical models used in the analyses for each car size group in Table 6: –

For the all injury severities risk: –

$$Y_{jkmnp} = \mu + B_j + C_k + E_m + F_n + (B*C)_{jk} + (E*F)_{mn} + M_p + e_{jkmnp},$$

where the effects are represented as above and by: –

$(B*C)_{jk}$	Interaction effect between type of object hit and speed limit of road,
$(E*F)_{mn}$	Interaction effect between sex of driver and age of driver, and
M_p	Effect for model of car.

For the fatal or serious injury severity risk: –

$$Y_{jklmnp} = \mu + B_j + C_k + D_l + E_m + F_n + (B*C)_{jk} + (E*F)_{mn} + M_p + e_{jklmnp},$$

where the effects are represented as above and by: –

$(B*C)_{jk}$	Interaction effect between type of object hit and speed limit of road,
$(E*F)_{mn}$	Interaction effect between sex of driver and age of driver, and
M_p	Effect for model of car.

24